# THE SCIENCE OF WELL-BEING

# THE SCIENCE OF WELL-BEING

*Happiness Hacks for a Fulfilling Life*

GIDEON RAYBURN

QuillQuest Publishers

# CONTENTS

# CHAPTER 1

# Introduction

Research in social psychology, particularly in the sub-field known as "Positive Psychology", has made waves with large sample sizes and longitudinal tests, making the possibility of well-being a reality. Most well-known is the 12-week happiness course introduced to Yale University by Laurie Santos. Comparing two equal-sized groups, one that completed the course and one that did not, it was discovered that the Happy Life Course did indeed increase happiness and fulfillment. These researchers, and Santos, offered a list of activities that rival the list of positive interventions. However, their activities were also published in an unappealing format: the mass of text intimidated potential users. Participants may be hesitant to fully engage with this course in the long-term for various reasons. Finally, the course demands funds that may not be available. Instituting an updated, dynamic, multimodal, and free list of survey-endorsed well-being effects with activity instructions sticks to be the natural progression in a field rich with knowledge about how to increase happiness.

According to the World Health Organization, the number one source of health-related suffering is depression. In fact, depression is projected to advance to the number one most common disability in the world by 2030. At the very least, health and happiness have a reciprocal relationship: being healthy makes us happier, and being happy makes us healthier. In order to combat the impending epidemic of depression and promote optimal physical, psychological, and social health, we need evidence-based solutions to increase well-being. However, participants often deviate from our 25 scientifically tested activities, usually for these three reasons: performing an act-of-kindness intervention for 1 week was found to only raise well-being for adolescents who both actively completed the activities, and for adults, 2 months was required to see a significant change in well-being via a gratitude visit; and selecting strengths and using them daily for 1 week increased happiness in the short-term, but well-being significantly increased after 3 weeks.

# CHAPTER 2

# Understanding Happiness

To avoid these problems, Lykken and Tellegen made use of the principle of hedonism. That is, they conducted research with approximately 4,000 twins from Minnesota, asking about their general life satisfaction, whether they consider themselves happier today than they were five years ago or ten years ago. They proposed that what we want when we seek to increase our happiness or the life satisfaction of other people is to increase our general well-being—our pleasant feelings about life on the one hand and our dissatisfaction on the other hand.

People wonder many things about happiness. What is it? What causes it to increase or decrease? Can we really increase our own happiness, or the happiness of others? One of the main conclusions in psychology in recent decades is that if we search for the answer to any of these questions, we first find psychology has a definition issue. For many, the word connotes hedonism—simply a focus on pleasure—while others associate it with broader feelings of life satisfaction and meaning. It is difficult for us to measure the extent of moral and pro-social behavior of people who were not alive 200 years ago. Therefore, the independent variables that truly influence the well-being of our species are lacking. Furthermore, there are difficulties in knowing which variables may have a great generality across the species or in studying the causal changes over time.

# CHAPTER 3

# Factors Influencing Well-Being

Think of transformative decisions as '4-D' (they involve four unique elements: duration-dependent dynamics underdetermined by available data), and of day-to-day decisions as resembling more tractable 3-D choices. Research on affective forecasting has established that people are not particularly talented at predicting their future feelings (specifically, emotional states) after transformative decisions, and this is what makes them risky. A simple-minded adaptation to avoid trade-offs would be to avoid risk and all transformative decisions altogether, and just focus on making the daily choices that, according to the painful decision-making process described above, should be less risky. But it's not that simple because transformative decisions, especially those that involve happiness (or the lack thereof) trigger longer-lasting and wider-ranging effects. If day-to-day decisions are nearsighted, transformative decisions have long-ranging implications, particularly related to well-being over time. Given our human nature, our lives are replete with choices and events that entail value transformations of the type that generate long-ranging effects on well-being. These can involve major trans-formations, such as the birth of a child, but also more quotidian matters, such as changes to whether we make day-to-day choices ourselves or from substantive (values-based), choices implemented by the self or others.

In an informative post for the blog 80,000 Hours, the ethics and public policy professor L.A. Paul draws a simple distinction between two kinds of life decisions: day-to-day decisions and trans-formative decisions. Day-to-day decisions are the routine choices we make from the menu of options that make up our daily lives: what to eat, how to spend our free time, what to wear, and so on. Transformative decisions are different: they are choices that lead us into lives that, in terms of opportunities, beliefs, desires, and values, are different from those we currently lead. Examples include leaving a job to travel the world, moving to another country, or getting married. Transformative decisions are risky because we don't know what our transformed lives will be like, and since we have no similar past experiences to help us predict the outcomes, we can't rely on introspection to assess the impact of such decisions. Day-to-day choices – at least those involving preferences familiar to us, such as a passion for salmon or a love of Shakespeare – appear less risky.

## CHAPTER 4

# Cultivating Positive Emotions

Deliberately increasing the experience of awe and wonder provides another effective happiness hack. Awe is an emotional response to something vast that is transcendent and does not fit into one's current mental structures. This sense of wonder often generates deeper interest in the world, personal improvement, and greater happiness. Awe shifts people from a narrow, self-focused state to a more generous, self-transcendent state and provides the opportunity to then build social connections facilitated by gratitude. Consider viewing more of nature, encouraging curiosity and exploration in yourself and others, and favoring experiences over possessions, to cultivate awe and wonder in your own life.

Positive emotions are beneficial when they broaden our cognition and action repertoires and build physical, intellectual, and social resources. To use the "broaden-and-build" theory of emotions, we can deliberately use happiness hacks that cultivate specific positive emotions. Cultivating gratitude is a powerful happiness hack. People who actively think and write about the things for which they are grateful experience more positive emotions, feel more connected to others, have stronger immune systems, are more likely to help others, and are generally happier. One effective practice is a gratitude journal in which you regularly write down things for which you are grateful. Establishing a consistent, long-term gratitude practice is most important, even if that means writing in your journal only once or twice a week.

# CHAPTER 5

# Building Meaningful Relationships

Lesson 1: The master of what makes life meaningful is simple: Joy does not exist in a vacuum. Understanding your overall happiness is not significant for your connection with other people. Which friendship surpasses Facebook friends? Cook concluded, "The information suggests that you have a limited virtual relationship with your friends, and that social support is not only due to people's attitudes. It is important for people's well-being and it is a valuable friend. Sometimes that stress is more important than a partner because friends are okay." Fixing a mobile network over concerns of old age well-being is a good idea. It is a known fact that if you are ill and a friend is worried, you will be friends with a dear person who has been with you in the time of need. "Cook said it's more than fine, but people don't talk about it."

Positive relationships are a keystone of happiness. People with close friendships and family are happier than those without. But it isn't enough to call or visit family and friends from time to time, Cook says. Quality counts. Your 20 best friendships trump 750

Facebook friends, she explains. Having a few close friend relationships is only second to our romantic partnerships in important relationships.

# CHAPTER 6

# Pursuing Personal Growth

It's common for people to get to a point in their lives and realize they're doing things to impress people they don't like. When you succeed and celebrate your own successes, you're feeding your reason to be, growing your willpower, and setting the stage for increased personal success. Have you ever been stuck in traffic and noticed how people respond to your gestures when you let them? Humans are deeply connected because we're part of a society and each individual plays a role in shaping the collective experience. When you're kind to someone or when someone is kind to you, the effects are felt throughout your community. So, they extend to whomever you interact with during the day. Additionally, people start repaying each other's kindness, so your direct and indirect kindness will come full circle to benefit you in the long run.

We're always evolving. So, it's important to be intentional about the kind of person we want to become. According to experts, there are four challenges that, when completed, give you the most satisfaction and happiness for the longest period of time. Take a few times each year to reflect on your life progress and what you can do to be a better version of yourself. You're rediscovering old favorites and learning new things you find exciting because learning and experimenting help keep life's magic alive. Continued curiosity throughout life helps you become more competent and powerful and boosts your self-esteem and excitement for the future.

# CHAPTER 7

# Practicing Gratitude

What are you most grateful for? There is no wrong answer. Act right in the moment, not just in general. Train your brain to savor the positive when you experience it. Let life's delights register in your brain. Make a single moment richer – a delectable meal, a shared laugh, a raucous kiss. Be mindful of them and engage. Have a good experience? Then savor it – and share it. Engage with a group of friends and do something kind for them. In psychology, "savoring" is the capacity to appreciate, relish, and luxuriate in positive experiences. Instead of letting the moment pass as if it was any other blip, savoring means living in the moment and heightening the positive experience. When we savor, our attention focuses like a laser beam on the joy we are experiencing (not away or on a cellphone), and this intensity makes joyful experiences more memorable. Savoring intensifies and lengthens the pleasure we derive from the positive moment, and this extension expertly slows time so the experience is enriched. If we savor these instances of love, joy, laughter, empathy, and passion, we can actually hold onto them and from a brain-wired view, make our lives and relationships last longer.

Our brains are hardwired to be sociable, ethical, and cooperative. Neuroscience research shows that the vagus nerve is key to the connected life because it slows our heart rate to synchronize with others and create "neural wi-fi." Altruistic behavior releases the pleasure neurochemical dopamine, so we are literally wired to help others. Magnetic Resonance Imaging data during moral reflection finds that the prefrontal-limbic network in the brain is especially goaded by values that reflect caring connections with others. Neuroscience shows that the more we sacrifice for others, the more we flourish. This is what Darwin called "survival of the kindest."

# CHAPTER 8

# Nurturing Physical Health

It is no coincidence that the science of well-being often includes a study of physical health. On the first day in a science of well-being class, students complete an in-class survey on many different aspects of health. These disclosures make that class like no other: profound gratitude is expressed for the simplest things, like having foot space under the desk. Why gratitude? Deep reverence for physical health underlie these thunderous disclosures of gratitude in health. Since health is integral to our happiness, it has no wonder that students express a deep appreciation of being free of illness and disease. Health is wealth and we take baking and inhaling sweet-smelling bread for granted. Earlier societies recognized local bakeries for providing what we consider today, an essential component of health.

The mechanisms underlying the mind's influence over biological systems have been called "psychosomatic." Reflexive associations between hedonism and health lead to the robust finding that subjective well-being. "That a human being should sacrifice him- or herself for the happiness of others is undoubtedly a high ideal. Unfortunately,

15

there can be another side to that ideal: that everyone should make the happiness of his fellowmen the sole object of life." Good things come to those who focus on the well-being of others, including caring for ourselves. On a plane descending into Miami, a flight attendant gave us the standard safety instructions and finished by saying, "put the oxygen mask on yourself before assisting others." Teachings that are often learned the hard way.

# CHAPTER 9

# Finding Balance in Life

Good company life initiatives, for instance, could encompass career development programs, stress management training, and stress control seminars, among other things. Proper supportive individual programs, notably those that recognize the venerable individuality of someone, can consist of adequate work-free periods; time to connect with family and community or even time for personal interests. Individuals should also include diverse activities away from work after work, weeklong as well as weekend social (or alone) responsibilities, particularly to people less privileged.

Research and experience suggest that workability and unworkability factors often interrelate with personal and organizational skills. Positive psychologists have also contributed to a growing understanding of the subject. In his 2004 book, "Authentic Happiness," Martin Seligman identifies three Roads to Happy Lives: The Pleasant Life, The Good Life, and The Meaningful Life. These three approaches (as being positive emotions and pleasures, engagement, and finding meaning) can be applied to practically any field, including this complex, multi-faceted research area of work-life balance. Researchers have also constructed models that can be used by both individuals and organizations to measure and assess outcomes of significant influencing factors. Such constructs are also essential to evaluating strengths that might be significant to counter job and personal stress. Often missed in research or not researched at all are the respective thoughts expressed by employees and employers about significant areas of balance in life.

As 21st-century living becomes busier and busier, maintaining balance in life is becoming more challenging. For the last decade, work-life balance as a topic has commanded a lot of attention from both individuals and organizations. A prominent contributing factor seems to be the ease of accessibility to technology combined with continuous employee engagement expectations. The trend in 2020 is that people are enticed to keep up with new lifestyle trends, making it essential for places of work and practitioners to gain insight to improve the quality of life.

# CHAPTER 10

# Managing Stress and Anxiety

For people who have severe anxiety and "calming" activities don't work, experts suggest the best alternative is to take your attention away from the situation and focus on a "cognitively engaging task." Think of balancing a checkbook, working on a crossword or Sudoku puzzle, or knitting. Doug says to make it a task that captivates your attention and as I mentioned above, it can't leave room for negative thoughts. If possible, when you are really feeling anxiety, share a moment with someone you feel comfortable with. I know in many cases, my dinner with friends in Sicily brought relief and according to many studies, talking to someone face-to-face can bring an outpouring of positive thoughts and memories. And Doug knows this from firsthand experience because he's observed it, not just others, but with his anxious dog who is happiest around him and his wife. Have the person offer input if possible to help solve problems and offer any positive reminders. This may go without saying, but just avoid pretending to be happy.

Explore stress-response apps and tech to chill out. Finally, the answer to the question should really start with the mind and influencing it to treat hard times like challenges instead of stressors. For years, it has been known that the mind is powerful and it can influence how the body responds to stressors. As humans evolved, stress was mainly due to "short-term physical activity," but chronic stress wasn't a thing. But the basic concept is if a person views a stressor as something that causes panic, the person develops a stress response and there is more of a negative impact on the body as well as an imbalance in the immune system. Understandably, when a person experiences positive emotions, there is an "undoing" of the stress response and immune system balance is restored. I'm no stranger to anxiety and here are some suggestions that I know have worked for me: Not surprisingly, I love yoga and meditation but when I can, I watch my dog, Daisy, taking in all the joy of being alive and suddenly, stress just isn't as bad.

# CHAPTER 11

# Enhancing Resilience

If we have a growth mindset, we are much more apt to be resilient and to recover from the negative events that unfold in our lives. Stanislawski (2017) writes, "Individuals who can remain hopeful and are able to control their negative emotions, are those who are more likely to experience traumatic growth." Everyday resilience is all about growth, about that second bounce, about being able to change and get stronger as time moves forward. There is an old Buddhist adage that no one deserves praise simply for observing the rising sun; we receive praise for our contributions to the world. Just the same, no one should feel bad about breaking when the world gets heavy and tough; we should all practice resilience and praise it only when we're out of that difficult, dark place, when we see a second sunrise. Resilience – our second bounce – will mature us and transform us. It's then that we've earned admiration and respect from our own selves, and from the world. We are strong by practicing these ten strategies that we have discussed.

Resilience is the ability to cope in the face of adversity – to survive, to keep going, and to bounce back from situations that you thought were going to sink you. Since hard times are unfortunately a part of life, it's important to hone resilience in our lives. Hofmann (2003) argues that relationships are the key to resilience, writing: "Social support is probably the most important and consistent predictor for resilience in adults. Good social relationships help people while they are coping with or recovering from stressful situations. If resilience is a survival skill, the best strategy for making use of this survival skill is when facing a horrendous life event is to engage with it: stay connected to others, lean on friends and family members, and remember that you are part of a community. Even when people are coping with highly traumatic events such as natural disasters, war, or domestic violence, actively seeking out social support can lead to positive changes (Tugade, Fredrickson, & Feldman Barrett, 2004)."

# CHAPTER 12

# Fostering Mindfulness

Theoretically, when you focus on being mindful, you can continue to remain fixated on the idea at hand and diminish interference from unrelated stimuli. As a result, mindfulness is associated with a plethora of cognitive improvements in the realm of inhibitory and higher frontal processes. One of the most well-documented theories regarding meditation and cognitive processes suggests that meditation increases self-regulation and focused concentration, two perspective qualities of attention. The PFC offers immediate top-down regulation of sensory cortices (related to neural synchrony) by enhancing communication and local circuit mechanisms to promote synchronous neural activity and attentional processes. Although these mechanisms and activations lend themselves to cognitive enhancement, mindfulness may particularly enhance deficits associated with aging or attentional maladies by targeting these mechanisms and enhancing attentional focus or control.

Raising and maintaining mindfulness is the goal of mindfulness meditation, which goes beyond just the minutes you are meditating. You continue to carry your mindfulness throughout the day and throughout life. The purpose of practicing mindfulness in this way is to increase your awareness and comprehension of whatever you are faced with. A quality and consciousness, mindfulness goes hand in hand with imagination. It has been suggested, and seems plausible, that the contemplative process often referred to in meditation and termed "mindfulness" by the Buddha was largely a function of the PFC. Recalling information or ideas while in a meditative state (both cognitive benefits of mindfulness or meditative practice) could mention the participation of various heteromodal association areas (integration areas) of the superior parietal cortex as well as PFC; and their recruitment in this process probably leads to increased top-down regulation and diminished cognitive interference, and would thus help to account for improvements in tasks requiring fronto-parietal function, whether in the realm of creativity, intelligence, or cognitive control.

# CHAPTER 13

# Engaging in Flow Activities

Everyone loves comparison shopping; years of advertising success reinforces how great it feels to get a trendy new gadget or the newest version of something you already have, especially when we know our friends are paying attention. Like a honeymoon phase, the novelty of our fresh purchase will boost our happiness for a short time, but this takes a U-shaped curve and soon we return back to our flat existence on our happiness floor, along with a credit card bill for the pleasure. To increase daily joy, avoid backsliding by curbing the need to compare possessions such as flashy new things. Teach yourself the habit of realizing social comparisons feedback on our innate desire to show higher status and can lead to lower self-care, envy, and a constant search for what else will bring us closer to the ever-dangling carrot of completeness. Alas, although we are prone to jealousy, changing our mindset about competition could help against these feelings.

"Flow" is that mental state when you are totally immersed in whatever you are doing. It often feels like time flies, and the world outside of whatever you are doing doesn't matter. One refreshing aspect about flow is that it often leads to a sense of great accomplishment and skillfulness and can make everything feel more meaningful. Everyone's flow looks different; for me, it is reading and writing blogs. For others, it may be playing a musical instrument or practicing a sport. To foster more flow into your life, seek that activity with just the right balance of difficulty and demand. A task too easy will lead to boredom, while a task too hard will cause anxiety. Even better, pursue those peak experiences, whenever possible, in presently engaging positively with one person, transporting yourself through nature or time period, or fully being in the moment with open awareness practicing mindfulness.

# CHAPTER 14

# Seeking Purpose and Meaning

If some of these directions weren't applicable, you just tell us you don't want to do that exercise—even though the procedure included this step or contained a video for another participant. When we compared participants following a similar plan for five days in a row, our mechanical Turk version had the added component of writing a 140-character vignette about your days. Most possible having more time slots for writing motivates action and distraction. Once or on taking control of the narrative that centers around stories that follow your most primary values. We also looked at ways of changing some pernicious habits and other participants strength based or the building activities, not surprisingly, were more effective.

On two of the days, not back to back, recall three positive experiences and then ask yourself why you think they happened in order to instill meaning. On a third day write a vignette about what you want to be remembered for. Who or what will be impacted by your being in the world? On the fourth day choose from a bank of 60 of the most important values or virtues. The best version of life will include various ratios of these, so finally choose your top ten. Ratchet those into an order that makes sense to you.

Purpose and meaning. What a granter of happiness! Active participants in one of our original studies focused their life around their most important values and their well-being increased. That makes sense—the areas of living that you invest in appreciate. So, here are some exercises to help you define, clarify, and pursue your purpose. Set aside 15 minutes a day for one of these exercises and learn your values:

# CHAPTER 15

# Setting and Achieving Goals

Our goal-setting mechanisms are highly unique. Still, most of us engage in raising or implementing such systems without ever wondering just how custom-built these mechanisms can truly be. Our hopes and imaginations could create a set of self-imposed goals in the future. Challenging goals set and obtained during or after this self-imposed period then offer the key experience that is activated, with ramifications for well-being adding from the emotional benefits of gratitude.

Gratitude for what we have is beneficial, but there are other tangible ways in which gratitude works to increase well-being by strengthening the emotions that arise, for example, when we are setting new goals or making progress on old ones, or for the future activities the accomplishment of new goals will make possible. By heightening the intensity or length of time of the positive emotions these moments evoke, gratitude ensures that these emotions are of a type that adds more to the overall happiness of our lives.

Gratitude – appreciating what we have – is at the center of many teachings, spiritual and secular. We often think of gratitude as being thankful for what's good in our lives, but when we set and achieve goals, we are grateful for our abilities to do this thing, such as being able to find work, accomplish work-related goals, or improve the circumstances of our work in general.

Setting and achieving goals in school, work, or life – for example, finding a job, increasing your income, getting better grades, or making new friends – are important for happiness. The key, though, is to set ourselves up for success by first selecting realistic goals and then working with purpose and drive to actually accomplish them. Goals add purpose to our lives, and that's very important for well-being.

# CHAPTER 16

# Embracing Optimism

In this book, the author shared dozens of practices designed to help you kick-start your well-being improvement, while only implicitly referring to their underlying scientific discovery. This book making these discoveries explicit has had the additional obvious advantage of detailing precise instructions for each technique. However, unexplained practices invite skepticism. And worse, they handicap ability to recast them as new ones, better suited to your needs. To overcome this self-restricting phenomenon, we herein investigate the science behind the practices. We start by avoiding the nomenclature of well-being elements and the metrics of psychology. We visually steer clear of subjective metrics.

The author looks at the power of different kinds of goals to help you live a fulfilling life and examines how our learning biases can show us paths to happiness. As you learn more about these biases, you will see that well-being is not an elusive or unattainable goal. It is instead a simple and innate mental skill that you can develop greatly with practice. You'll discover six aphorisms that reveal clear paths you can take to improve your own and others' well-being. Once you apply all these tools, you will reach the extraordinary realization that well-being is the skill that slowly turns every challenge, difficulty, imperfection, impermanence, hardship, inadequacy, and even tragedy into an opportunity for a crucial cognitive exercise, one that leads to enduring, ever-growing happiness.

# CHAPTER 17

# Developing
# Self-Compassion

Another technique researchers developed to cultivate self-compassion involves writing exercises. You can benefit from the exercises for those days when you criticize yourself and feel the pressure of external demonstrations. Using phrases such as "I am enough", "I am worthy of love", "I care for myself and others", which serves to remind the support that surrounds you and targets self-criticism. One exercise that is a particularly powerful self-compassionate tool is a letter writing exercise: write a letter to yourself from the perspective of a friend who loves you unconditionally. If you do that, recognize the friend's difficulties manifesting in your own shortcomings and promote self-understanding compassion, which lowers defense mechanisms and increases the level of anxiety, while compassion provides and encourages patient optimism.

If you could be friends with anyone in the world, would you choose someone who mistreated you or neglected you? Since it's clear that being kind towards oneself with discretionary intention is beneficial for us, let us now talk about how we can increase compassionate feelings and behaviors of self-compassion. If we want to be more self-compassionate towards ourselves, we need to stop being critical, judgmental, and extremely competitive. Challenge your negative thoughts: instead of giving yourself some negative evaluation, examine them for validity. Practice self-consoling if you find yourself in a difficult situation – instead of criticizing yourself as if you were a friend and you did the same to them – with a kind and empathic voice offering words telling yourself. One study showed that these voices in the process of compassion caused some people to become more resilient and more likely to share with others.

# CHAPTER 18

# Strengthening Emotional Intelligence

Emotional intelligence supports one's daily life in various ways. Emotional intelligence is associated with the ability to choose happiness not only for oneself but for others as well. People who experience life satisfaction tend to have better emotional understanding and competence. It has also been well-documented that individuals with high emotional intelligence scores are happier and have higher life satisfaction scores. This is especially true for individuals who attend enrichment programs; their life satisfaction scores are exponentially higher than average students. Higher emotional intelligence enables us to effectively cope with stress and gives us flexibility to adapt to different social situations. Students with high emotional abilities excel academically and have high self-esteem.

"Emotional intelligence is the ability to perceive, understand, manage, and use emotions." Emotional intelligence leads to successful social and personal interactions. Emotional intelligence comprises two areas: emotional ability and emotional competence. People who are high in emotional ability tend to be well-tuned with their emotions and the emotions of others, and tend to show more happiness and forgiveness. Conversely, emotional incompetence or inabilities, such as lacking emotional understanding and intelligence, are related to limitations in emotional knowledge. Emotional intervention is also one of the main aspects in guiding us to successful interpersonal skills in multiple levels of context.

# CHAPTER 19

# Promoting Work-Life Balance

Spread work over time. If, in order to get all the work done, you completely fill your working hours with various meetings and professional tasks, virtually every day, you are not alone. The problem with this kind of lifestyle is that for most people, it causes stress. A good hack is to take some time to consider how long it would take to complete the tasks that you have ahead of you. And, however improbable it might seem, you could create an agenda in which all the tasks are spread over the week on the very day you wake up. On Monday, you are creating and sending 15 invoices. On Tuesday, you are working on some presentation documents. On Wednesday, you're going to visit 6 clients and the day really is going to be easier than usual. No more than usual, there are going to be work to do. During the days, it is recommended to take several breaks to work efficiently when the coming challenges begin.

A 2015 survey showed that 70% of American workers just cannot manage to find a good balance between their work and personal life. And this is not just an American problem; across the world, a large percentage of professionals, entrepreneurs, and freelancers all feel that they are inadequate in managing the time dedicated to work and that dedicated to their personal stuff. If you suffer from the inability to balance work and personal life, here are 7 tools that will help you avoid workaholic burnout and will help you recover some precious personal time. It will also give you less stress, higher quality work, more personal satisfaction, and more success at work and in business.

# CHAPTER 20

# Creating a Supportive Environment

Many factors, and habit is one of them. By repeating a behavior, this behavior will require less and less cognition, therefore allowing us to accomplish this behavior more efficiently, and to use our mental resources on something else. Over time, our context will be configured by the habits we have adopted, therefore creating a reinforcing dynamic between the environment we evolve in and the habits we have developed. If we come back to the tree metaphor, behavioral habits cause recurring roads to be drawn in the original soil. These more and more borrowed roads eventually condense and harden to give birth to the road we will prefer to take.

Putting happiness on our to-do list goes a long way towards creating a supportive environment for ourselves and for the people around us. Our environment is like a tree, whose branches are the moral values that humans have exercised across time and across societies. Some values are cherished across many cultures throughout the centuries, while others are either evolutionary spills or something that emerges with socio-historical processes. Whatever the origin, most of the moral values that people share can be found along the branches of the tree. Together, these moral values form an important basis for our own moral compass. But with time, our moral compass might guide us in a different direction. There are many factors that influence this movement such as family, social circles, education, the media, or in general the context in which we evolve.

# CHAPTER 21

# Practicing Mindful Eating

Dr. Albers is also a chocolate connoisseur and believes that we should enjoy real chocolate, but not just grab the modern, medicinal bars and mindlessly eat to feel better. However, she disagrees with traditional Japanese custom of buying and eating chocolates as part of entertainment at the airport after travels. The greater awareness and engagement will transform the habitual eating and drinking of happiness to the fulfillment sought through mindful eating. What was the last time you practiced an everyday, routine activity with the focus of a Zen master? Relax and meditate on the action of drinking and eating. Allow enough time, purchase and cook real and healthy food and take time to experience the revitalized tastes. Go to the market on foot or by bicycle, holding no thoughts other than to pay that complete awareness and even reverence to the guardian of our health that is water, drink a glass daily. Focus on small ingredients' details, taking the time to mince vegetables, peel fruits, prepare sauces, understand this joy and sorrow implying all necessary gestures and so recognize the breath of the stress of life to the very act of life.

Do you want to unlock the happiness held in food? Dr. Albers is a psychologist who knows that pigging out on mood-altering foods such as chocolate blocks our taste buds to the complex happiness found in simpler, more nourishing dishes. She's a proponent of mindful eating, warning that if you gobble down too much comfort food such as chocolate, it turns off the taste buds. However, she added, "if you pull back and just savor a sliver of it, this is really what's going to help your taste buds become more reaccustomed to the flavors. When we do that, we become more aware of the subtler flavors in other things in our environment." According to a UC Davis news in a 2012 news release, "her three steps for mindful eating include "savoring, by slowing down, fully tasting and enjoying your food; turning off the autopilot and that nagging internal chatter; and reducing the guilt and frustration by accepting it, rather than focusing on those unwanted feelings."

# CHAPTER 22

# Exploring Mind-Body Connections

Exploring mind-body connections should not be about establishing the superiority of relaxation techniques over moderate or vigorous exercise; the question is not 'What is the best type of exercise?' Instead the question is 'What is the best type of exercise for a particular target population or individual?' Results of the studies in both ordered-exercise and self-referred exercises suggest that it is not yoga, but a physical postural exercise that people engage in, Regardless of which exercise regimen one has a preference for, the important question is: "How do we harness the power of relaxation practices, engage in moderate or vigorous exercise, and continue to practice purposeful acts of kindness and altruistic behavior?"

Basic research into mind-body interventions is leading to a fuller understanding of health and well-being. Some nine hours of mindfulness meditation training can help to mitigate psychological stress, and neuroscience research provides a clearer picture of the effects of meditation training on the brain, offering a more complete description of the underlying brain mechanism that may lead to the development of more-targeted meditation programs. Consistent neuroscience reports of mindfulness-modulating brain circuits and reducing pain and pain-related unpleasantness have been paralleled by behavioral evidence that mindfulness enhances complicated cognitive skills and that an 8-week training in mindfulness meditation was associated with structural changes in the brain. In particular, mindfulness meditation was posited to target task-set reconfiguration mechanisms and contingency detection. Further research is beginning to link mindfulness training to slower cognitive decline and brain aging, which suggests that mindfulness training programs may hold promise for aging.

Mind-body interventions focus on the interactions among the brain, mind, body, and behavior, and on ways to use the mind to change the body and promote health and well-being. Changing the directionality of the relationship assumed to exist between the mind and body can lead to intriguing spin-offs in health benefits. For instance, people in the United States who feel luckier exercise more, quit smoking more easily, and are more likely than others to seek help in difficult times. In tough times, such as when recovering from cardiac surgery, people who feel luckier may actually be luckier in a material way. If feeling luckier or even acting luckier can improve health and well-being, finding ways to purposefully inculcate a 'lucky attitude' could lead to the identification of simple, inexpensive ways to harness the power of such placebo-like optimism for health promotion and disease prevention.

# CHAPTER 23

# Harnessing the Power of Meditation

More Happiness Meditation seems to create lasting happiness. A study that followed people who had just finished a three-month meditation retreat found enduring improvement in outcomes. This was regardless of meditation style chosen by the individuals. Consistent with these findings from a retreat, another study showed that attending weekly meditation practices for six weeks led to increased TLC and sense of kindness toward others. Other studies have had people doing daily sessions for as little as a week or two. They still saw significant increases in their felt compassion and well-being.

Have you been thinking about doing some meditation but haven't got started yet? The advantage of meditation has been known for centuries. Recent scientific research is identifying more and more benefits. If you're wanting to learn how to meditate, there is a free resource. It has detailed instructions on several different forms of meditation. And it has a side-by-side tool where you can compare different approaches. Here are just a few reasons why you might want to give it a try.

# CHAPTER 24

# Finding Joy in the Present Moment

Deci and Ryan found that human motivation is based on three needs: relatedness, autonomy, and competence. For those of you who have been following all along, you might remember that Deci and Ryan's Self-Determination Theory is also intricately tied to long-term happiness and fulfillment, similar to well-being motivation. Let's take, for example, chasing a sunset. Reflecting on the beauty as well as being in the present moment would help in cultivating happiness. Welcome to part three of the six-part series on the science of happiness. Since we now know that the brain is built to prioritize survival over happiness and that it automatically finds things to worry about, we need to find openings. The most direct way into our happy place is this – being present.

On a basic level, doing new things with people we care about gives us a burst of joy. It's also what helps us form strong relationships with others. In other words, the last time you chatted with a friend over ice cream or saw a movie with your partner, the quality time was shaping your brain for the better. Also, with new experiences, we explore more opportunities for cultivating positive emotional experiences, which is a key component of overall happiness. Exercise makes us happy not just because we get a mood boost, but also because it contributes to long-term happiness. Warm fuzzies are fun, but lasting fulfillment and satisfaction come from fostering a sense of meaning in the activities we do.

# CHAPTER 25

# Cultivating Resilient Thinking

Disclaimer: There are courses that can help you develop a better mental tension on this topic, such as The Science of Well-Being, The Yale Happiness certificate, TED Talks on Mental Health, Fear Setting, Resilience, or even guided meditations specifically designed for anxiety, stress, or depression that can be found anywhere on the internet. However, I am not a psychologist, doctor, or psychiatrist, so it is best to consult your peers before trying out any new method in case you have never given them a go before or if you start feeling a little strange after using some of the methods below. If some of these simply don't feel right and exacerbate your anxiety, stress, or depression, be them moderate or severe, it is best to stop using them, as everyone is different and, because of this, one person may find a science-supported method that has changed their life, and someone else may find that the same method can sometimes influence their mood in a different direction. Ever given something a go or wanted to test something that you believe may better combat such uninvited guests? Then tell us in the comments section below how it went.

I still remember the exact day when I was diagnosed with Generalized Anxiety Disorder. I was sitting once again at the therapist's office, with this time an "Oh no!" internship around the corner as opposed to an "Oh no!" final test. This dress rehearsal of a mental chess match that I was playing with myself was wearing me down and, no matter what strategies, tips, and tricks we could conjure up, it seemed that resilience is not the most forthcoming of friends when it is most needed. Thankfully, that has changed over time. And it's not like the external circumstances that were most fear-inducing have subsided or have become easier to deal with. It's just that I've learned from the connections of psychologists, professors, and happiness experts—through platforms like Positive Psychology studies or TED talks—on emotional resilience. And today I invite you to join me on this list of 25 Science-Backed Tools for Cultivating Resilient Thinking in a contemporary society that seems too often to feed on stress, anxiety, and depression.

# CHAPTER 26

# Improving Sleep Quality

Social cognitive theory suggests that certain self-regulatory mechanisms are important for implementing health behavior. In this study, these mechanisms were applied to the behavior of sleep enhancement to examine their relationship with sleep quality. The study involved college students who completed questionnaires, diaries, and actigraphic recordings over a period of seven nights. The results of the analysis showed that many of the hypothesized indices were significantly related to improved sleep quality and reduced wake-time after sleep onset. However, the relationship between behavior at the beginning of the semester and sleep quality at the end of the semester was not significant. This suggests that the challenges associated with implementing these behaviors may not be fully understood or accounted for by current behavior theory. The study proposes extensions to the model to better understand the role of self-regulatory behavior change mechanisms in promoting health-enhancing behaviors.

# CHAPTER 27

# Enhancing Social Connections

Given this data, perhaps we should not be surprised that connecting one-on-one with a genuine shared human experience can lead to a significant increase in group performance. When Basecamp CEO and co-founder Jason Fried experimented with a different presentation style, a shift in his company's performance gave noticeable effects far beyond the usual benefit a new inspiring speaker tends to bring. In fact, over 40% of the audience rated Jason's talk at Ignite Chicago conference as the best one he has given. At Torley, the product manager Jason has worked with applies the teaching technique of the late Carnegie Mellon professor Randy Pausch, putting intimate anecdotes to explain the concepts behind the software packages they place in the hands of new college hires, as well as experts who are continuing to mentor one another. Having been raised in Finland and being less emotionally expressive in conversations, I asked Jason to elaborate on the details of his conversation strategy when he told me about his mentoring style during the daily standups.

"The quality of our relationships matters - it affects everything from games on a computer to succeeding at a rhyming competition or playing a novel game." This was the conclusion of MIT associate professor and renowned psychologist Alex "Sandy" Pentland. To uncover the specifics of what fosters stronger social relationships, Pentland gave different groups tags with tracking devices to monitor the way they interacted. He discovered that a group's ability to communicate in balance or take turns led to increased social ties. Interestingly, the richness of the content or conversation itself did not seem to matter and it was simply the "give and take" during conversation that led to more connected groups. Pentland also discovered patterns in body language and posture that added to the richness of these interactions.

# CHAPTER 28

# Fostering a Sense of Belonging

There is merit to this approach for different reasons. First, social connections established around a shared passion are more meaningful than those that emerge from shared geographic location. This is why people feel so good when a sports team wins – they feel connected to one another through team allegiance. Second, in the long run, being with people who care about things that you do is more satisfying. While some people like living a solitary life, people who have 2 or 3 friends at work, people who belong to a PTA, garden, or another special interest group, report being happier than those who do not, even with other important factors statistically controlled. When I first started teaching courses at Eastern Washington University on Positive Psychology, students often asked me why the field had so many studies that suggested that if you do any one of a number of behaviors, you will become instantly happier.

A sense of social belonging is a need that is so basic that we feel emotional pain when it is not met. Yet, in spite of the importance of social connection in producing high levels of happiness, people in all stages of life join countless groups and organizations where these connections might occur and often sit alone staring at the TV or computer. There are many things that people can do to increase social connections. The first is to take advantage of our options. Think about joining organizations that reflect your values or interests. If you appreciate the arts, join a group that supports local theater or galleries. If you would like to be more active, join organizations that support causes you think are important like an environmental or political group. Maybe there is a religious, community, or sports organization that you could take advantage of. Whatever you choose, it should be relevant to what you care about or it likely won't satisfy your need for connection.

# CHAPTER 29

# Embracing Change and Uncertainty

What is practically useful about cultivating awe and wisdom to combat an entitlement mindset? "The remedy for an 'entitlement' mindset is gratitude." It fosters emotional and interpersonal resilience. Instead of giving in to one's "rightful indignation," an attitude of gratefulness helps us switch out of zero tolerance mode for mistakes and failures in others. It triggers a positive feedback loop where others respond to our grace with contributions and assurances of their competence, thereby enhancing resources of the neighborhood or collective. These become the invisible scaffolding that buttress our happiness by providing social support in stressful times; opportunities to admire, teach, and celebrate; and the ability to engage in meaningful and enriching endeavors.

Change is inevitable, but our discomfort with uncertainty often keeps us stagnant. That's why we try to "fix" our lives without pausing and evaluating whether the changes we seek are progress or merely changes. Knowledge and experience may help us foster a greater level of comfort with an uncertain world. But true wisdom may not be found through mathematical or vocational expertise. It may, instead, require reacquainting ourselves with the wonders of nature's web of life. It reminds us that we are not petulant passengers on Planet Earth, but simply rare beneficiaries of its harmony and life-supporting infrastructure. Suddenly, awe reemerges.

# CHAPTER 30

# Promoting Self-Care

Despite the fact that one of the lessons of positive psychology is that a high degree of satisfaction in one's home life is critical for happiness, not everyone will have perfect home lives. Children may have developmental challenges, spouses may fall ill, young family members may succumb to debilitating conditions. It is because of the existence of such crises and challenges that we need a theory-based, strategic plan for our own well-being. This is true regardless of career position. In short, our private, personal lives are both our primary source of energy and our primary laboratory for positive inhabitation. From there, we can extend leadership in positive institutions as well.

Well-being refers to a state of feeling well in the most complete sense. This includes the very basic physical sensation of feeling hunger or pain, to the ability to sustain and enjoy nurturing relationships with loved ones. Flow is a transcendent state of deep absorption while doing something that stretches us and employs our full capacity. Self-care is one straightforward way in which people can address and remediate vulnerabilities in their well-being. It is a well-known maxim that humans need to maintain their physical and psychological health if they are serious about being creative warriors and agents of change, even if they don't understand the science of why this is the case.

# CHAPTER 31

# Embracing Vulnerability

Marry yourself. And all this while, this uncertain phenomenon - self-equality, contentment, love - all has to do with life. It is what we aim to achieve from life. Not one citizen of this world would deny wanting joy. Therefore, you. You are the person who should matter the most to you. Does happiness from others' perception have to be a constant trial? Rediscover love for yourself. Perhaps catchy poetry or a frustratingly structured 7-beat sentence. Remain honest with your insights. Writing think inefficiency is like losing something before it is actually gone, I wrote. Dig deeper. Why should a solitary room only echo pain? I want my silent repose in the emptiness that reverberates my only company to also feel my happiness. After all, wonderful things do accompany the feeling as well. Find yourself in another, and feel yourself fill all corners and reach all edges of imagination and reality. Speak to yourself, you need it. Alone times are, after all, times when we are able to listen to ourselves better.

Accept that there will be uncomfortable situations in life. Surround yourself with unpleasant situations. Look at things dispassionately. We may like or not like something, but if we do establish that we are in no position to alter the situation, we may realize, well, feeling either way, the event, and life, will keep going on. Seeing the bigger picture can be calming. Understanding life to have its ups and downs and that one cannot ensure it not to happen is another comfort.

Make room. Your fear will not go easily, so make room for it. Keep living your life with that uncomfortable feeling beside you. This will do two things - it will make you sure that you have acknowledged fear and that it cannot act as a basis. It allows it to dissipate by not giving it any importance.

Acknowledge your fears. One way to shoo off fear is to embrace it every day. As your fear gets more concentrated, it dissipates. It is like shining light on a shadow. You must do this daily. To close your fear is to hide. Thus, the feeling becomes a part of you. Acknowledging that you have nothing to do in solving this fear is also important. You have acknowledged it, and that is the only way to use it. Fear is an emotion that appears when you start to question yourself. However, recognizing them and that this subject is of no importance keeps fear trapped in a box.

# CHAPTER 32

# Sustaining Well-Being in the Long Run

Mindfulness—more than any other mental habit—is the practice that conserves our meaning and well-being. When we are mindful, we relate to the elements that matter to us: nature, the cosmos and the divine. Above all, mindfulness allows us to experience life in its full vibrancy and visceral richness, taking delight in the wildness of our children, in the intriguing shapes of human ingenuity, in the astonishing variety of life forms that call this extraordinary planet home. And the power of hummingbird wings in motion is a gift of grace. If at times we forget our life is so miraculous, mindfulness permits us to touch the wonders of existence, reacquainting us with the preciousness of life. More than two thousand years ago, Aristotle wrote that the most fulfilling life is one in which we use our unique talents and attributes to serve humanity, thereby cultivating our personal and collective potential. The science of well-being validates Aristotle's idea—finding that serenity, happiness, flow, meaning, love, and personal satisfaction emerge when we cultivate virtue in the context of personal and collective meaning. The mental habits can be exercised individually or in concert with one another; focusing on one strength without neglecting the others may provide the most fulfilling and exhilarating route to long-term well-being. So - create, engage, love, protect, yearn, be, and savor. At the end, you will find a life well lived—and that is the ultimate human pursuit.

The last mental habit that helps sustain meaning and well-being in the long run is mindfulness. Mindfulness is defined as a state of being fully present in the moment, without judgment. Whether one is contemplating the true name of the Divine like Rumi, or simply marveling at a piece of fruit like Mary Oliver, mindfulness is the conduit by which we can savor life's small pleasures and touch the world's wondrous moments. The ability to pay attention to these moments immersed in present awareness is the key to foster a life of intimacy, fulfillment, and moral purpose. This ability to attune and connect can help us build bonds with loved ones, acquaintances, and ourselves. We can also use mindfulness to strengthen the attention muscle helping to fortify the mental habits discussed in this series of articles.

9 798330 588909